I0829868

The 20-Minute Miracle

How to Use Ozone Water to Promote
Good Health and Wellness in
People, Pets, and Plants

by Mike Casey

FIRST EDITION

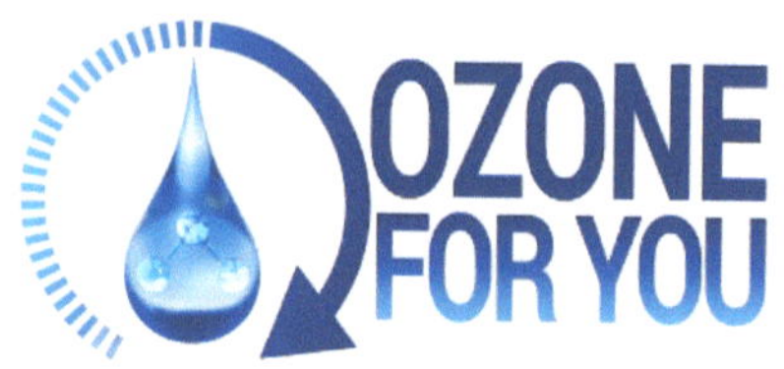

Copyright 2018 by Mike Casey

www.OzoneForYou.com

All rights reserved. No portion of this book may be reproduced - mechanically, electronically, or by any other means, including photocopying - without permission from the author.

NOTICE: All information, content, and material are for informational purposes only and are not intended to serve as a substitute for the consultation, diagnosis, and/or *medical* treatment of a qualified physician or healthcare provider. *MEDICAL* EMERGENCY If you have a *medical* emergency, call your doctor or 911.

Table of Contents

Dedication

This book is dedicated to all the people who needlessly suffer from bacterial and viral infections. It is my hope that this book finds its way into your hands.

Acknowledgements

I want to thank Bruce Hinkle, Chief Technical Officer of PureQuest Ozone Technologies, who introduced me to the miracle of Ozone Water and helped to make sure the facts in this book are true and correct. Bruce is one of the few experts in the field.

I also want to thank my wonderful wife, Joyce. I could not have authored and produced this book without her able assistance, support, and encouragement.

Glossary

Activated oxygen – Another name for ozone in water. See Ozone.

Allotropic – The ability of some chemical elements to exist in two or more different forms in the same physical state as *allotropes*. Graphite, charcoal, and diamond are allotropes of carbon.

Aerobic – Relating to, involving, or requiring oxygen.

Anaerobic – Relating to, involving, or requiring an absence of free oxygen.

Bacteria – A single-cell pathogen. A member of a large group of unicellular microorganisms that have cell walls but lack organelles and an organized nucleus, including some that can cause disease. Most common bacteria are anaerobic.

Bruise – Blood or bleeding under the skin that may or may not be due to trauma; typically black and blue at first, with color changes as healing progresses.

Cell lysis – Destruction of a cell by disintegration due to rupture of the cell wall or membrane.

Diffusion – The net movement of molecules or atoms from a region of high concentration to a region of low concentration. A result of random motion of the molecules or atoms.

Disinfection – The process of cleaning something in order to destroy bacteria.

Free Oxygen – Molecular oxygen available for respiration by organisms. Molecular oxygen is the oxygen molecule, (O_2), that is not connected with another element to form a compound.

Free radical – An uncharged molecule (typically highly reactive and short-lived) with an unpaired valence electron.

Half-life – The time required for any specific property to decrease by half.

Infection – The invasion of an organism's body tissues by disease-causing agents, their multiplication, and the reaction of host tissues to the infectious agents and the toxins they produce.

Inflammation – Part of the complex biological response of body tissues to harmful stimuli, such as pathogens, damaged cells, or irritants. A protective response involving immune cells, blood vessels, and molecular mediators. Five classic signs are: heat, pain, redness, swelling, and loss of function.

Osmosis – a process by which molecules pass through a semipermeable membrane from a less concentrated solution into a more concentrated one, thereby equalizing the concentrations on each side of the membrane.

Oxygen – A colorless, odorless reactive gas and a life-supporting component of air. A chemical element, atomic number 8, oxygen forms about 20% of the earth's atmosphere.

Ozone – An allotropic form of oxygen consisting of three oxygen atoms (O_3), also called activated oxygen when mixed into water. Formed by electrical discharges or ultraviolet light. Unstable, but not dangerous. Oxygen prefers to return to, and remain as, O_2. Ozone will return to O_2 in a short period of time at room temperature by casting off a free radical of oxygen (O_1).

Pathogen – Bacteria, virus, or other microorganism that can cause disease.

Passive diffusion – A movement of ions and other atomic or molecular substances across cell membranes without the need for energy input. The movement is from an area of high concentration to an area of low concentration.

Skin – The thin, semipermeable layer of tissue forming the outer covering of the body of a person or animal.

Sprain – A stretching or tearing of ligaments, the fibrous tissue that connects bones to joints.

Sterilization – The process of making something free of bacteria or other living microorganisms.

Virus – A single-celled infective agent typically consisting of a nucleic acid in a protein coat. Too small to be seen by light microscopy, a virus can multiply only within the living cells of a host.

Water – Colorless, odorless liquid can dissolve a variety of different substances. Water is called the "universal solvent" because it dissolves more substances than any other liquid.

Preface

The term *miracle* has been overused; however, not in the case of ozone water. When ozone is placed in water, it becomes *activated oxygen* and amazing things happen, but only for a short period of time. This is like Clark Kent turning into Superman, but for only twenty minutes. On a cellular level, ozone water acts as Superman in the fight against pathogens. It destroys 99.99% of all viruses and bacteria on contact. Pathogens have no defense against it. Ozone water dissolves bacteria and viruses' outer walls on contact in a process called *cell lysis*. The single-celled pathogens are effectively destroyed on contact and cease to exist, like a human body dropped into molten lava: here one second, gone the next. Ozone (O_3) throws off a free radical of oxygen (O_1) when it returns to its preferred state (O_2). This free-radical oxygen is highly reactive on a cellular level. After twenty minutes, ozone(O_3) returns to its preferred form(O_2). Superman turns back into Clark Kent, and disinfected surfaces remain disinfected. This battle against bacteria and virus has been won. The war continues. [1, 2, 3, 4]

This book attempts to change the focus and narrative from the controversy surrounding ozone gas to the benefits of ozone water. The benefits of ozone water are undeniable, government-approved, and organic, yet most Americans have never heard of them.

This book will educate you about the ways in which ozone water can benefit people, pets, and plants during the twenty minutes that activated oxygen remains activated. During that time, ozone water can help promote good health and wellness for people, pets, and plants in amazing ways.

You can now disinfect almost any surface, easily, safely and effectively. Think of the possibilities. If you are in a battle against bacteria, viruses, or mold, try ozone water. You can win the war against pathogens with "Superman" on your side.

Introduction to Ozone Water

– The World's Safest, Most Powerful Disinfectant

When ozone, the world's most powerful disinfectant, is added to water, the "universal solvent," the newly-formed ozone water becomes the world's safest and most powerful disinfectant, organically disinfecting almost any surface on contact.

- Ozone water destroys 99.99% of all bacteria and viruses on contact. [1,2,3,21]
- Ozone water is approved by the FDA, USDA Organic, and the EPA. [6,7,8,9]
- Ozone water is comprised only of activated oxygen (O_3) and water (H_2O). [3]
- 100% organic. (O_3H_2O). [3]
- Ozone water is easy and inexpensive to produce. [3]
- Ozone water kills pathogens by dissolving their body structure on contact. [1,2,3,4]
- Pathogens have no defense against ozone water. [1,2,3,4]
- Ozone water kills virus and bacteria 3,000 x faster than chlorine. [21]
- Ozone water leaves no residue. [3]

Historical note: Nickola Tesla patented the first ozone generator in 1896, and in 1900, formed the Tesla Ozone Company. His patented ozone generator was for medical use. One of his original units is still in working condition. [4]

What did Tesla, one of the world's greatest scientists, know?

Ozone water's disinfection abilities promote good health and wellness by helping to prevent infection, reduce inflammation, and promote rapid healing. Ozone water is not a cure; rather, it is preventative because it destroys bacteria and viruses before

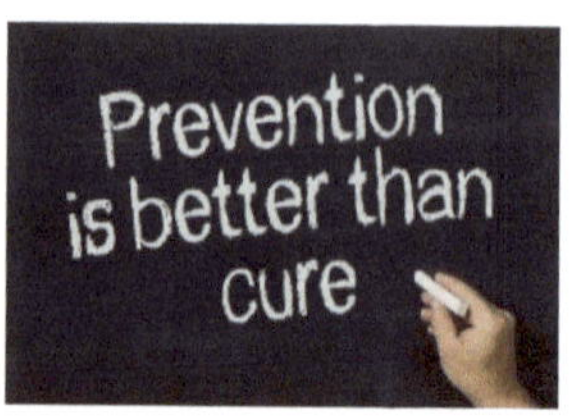

they can multiply and make you ill. Prevention is far better than cure, because it prevents the discomfort of becoming sick. It also saves the inconvenience and cost of medical treatment. [10,11,12,13]

Oxygen is the #1 essential ingredient for healing. It has been known since the 1850s that skin absorbs oxygen. Ozone water promotes rapid healing by providing a large amount of activated oxygen. Its high oxygen content oxygenates the skin by passive diffusion. The oxygen is then picked up by the blood and transported to the site of injury by the circulatory system. This activated oxygen provides the energy necessary for healing. [10,11,18]

More oxygen = less infection = faster healing.

There are two methods to produce ozone water. This book will detail how they can both be used together to help promote good health and rapid healing for people, pets, and plants.

1. Ozone-water faucets offer the convenience of ozone water on demand at your kitchen or utility sink.
2. An inexpensive bubble-stone ozone generator will produce ozone water in as little as five minutes. It can also be used to add additional ozone to water during applications and ozone-water immersion. It is portable and can be taken on travels for protection against pathogens on airplanes or in crowded spaces.

Ozone in water is called activated oxygen. While activated the oxygen molecule is free, ready, willing and able to promote rapid healing. Activation only lasts for a short period of time, then the activated oxygen returns to the normal state of oxygen. Once produced, ozone water must be used as soon as possible. Ozone water's disinfection abilities have a twenty-minute half-life at room temperature. The ability of ozone water to disinfect diminishes rapidly over time, and increased temperatures will also shorten ozone's life. Ozone (O_3) returns to the preferred form of oxygen (O_2) in a process that is 100% organic and leaves no residue. During this process, ozone casts off a free radical of oxygen (O_1) and becomes O_2. This free radical of oxygen is extremely powerful and beneficial to the human body.

Do not be confused by the 20-minute rule. Ozone water should be used within twenty minutes after it is produced, because ozone water's disinfection ability diminishes rapidly over time. The surfaces disinfected by ozone water will remain disinfected until a pathogen contacts the surface and begins to multiply. Applied once or twice daily, ozone water will disinfect surfaces and prevent pathogens from becoming multiplying into infectious colonies.

Higher quality of water will yield more highly ozonated water. Reverse osmosis (RO) water is better than tap water for producing ozone water; however, either will work. RO

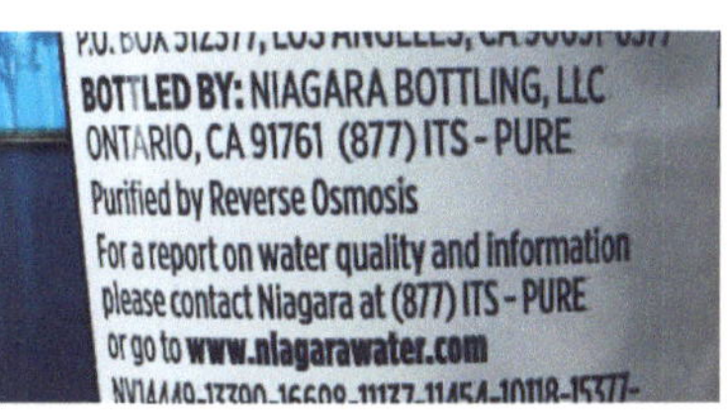

water can be found in any store that sells water. Read the label to confirm. In comparison, tap water will require a longer period of bubbling to reach a high level of ozone. The reason is that ozone will neutralize any organic material in tap water, like chlorine, before it will begin to increase the ozone content in the water. Tap water also has a higher level of dissolved solids that will be left behind when the ozone water evaporates. These dissolved solids may or may not be affected by the ozone.

Historical note: Ozone water evaporates faster than regular water.

If you are going to use a home RO water filtration unit for immersion or burn applications, check the total dissolved solids monthly. RO membranes are slowly destroyed by chlorine over a period of several years, so it is important to know if the unit is working properly if you use the RO water for ozone water applications. You can purchase a total dissolved solids (TDS) meter that easily checks your RO unit's functionality. Reverse osmosis should remove a minimum of 90% of the total dissolved solids of the incoming water. Adding an 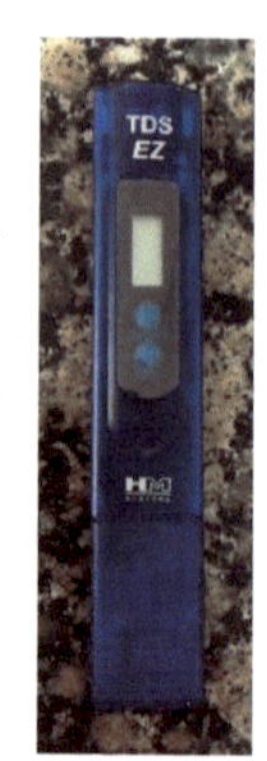 in-line carbon filter and changing the unit's prefilters regularly is important for long-term life of the RO membranes. If it has not been serviced regularly, there is a good chance that the RO unit is faulty. If the unit is not working properly, consider replacing it with an ozone faucet.

Ozone water is easy and inexpensive to make. It can be produced or placed in most clean containers. Glass and stainless steel containers are best; however, plastic will work just fine.

Historical note: The space race developed synthetic materials like Teflon. These synthetic, chemical-resistant materials were vital to the miniaturization of ozone generators and ozone faucets. [4]

Bubble-stone ozone generators should continue to be used during ozone water immersion. Adding ozone during ozone water immersion will keep ozone concentrations as high as possible.

If you have an ozone water faucet, use it to fill containers, then add bubble stone to continue to add ozone to the water. Remember, ozone dissipates over time, and upon contact with surfaces. Think of it like a can of soda. When the can is opened, it has lots of fizz, but after twenty minutes, there is very little fizz. The difference is that you can continue to bubble ozone to keep the "fizz" level high.

Use caution. Some portable ozone generators can produce enough ozone gas to irritate the lungs and make you cough. OzoneForYou.com offers small portable ozone generators that produce ozone gas under the OSHA threshold[5]

If you are sensitive to ozone gas, you can do several things to lessen the effect:

- Use a fan to disperse the gas.
- Place a carbon mask over your mouth and nose.
- Keep the room well-ventilated.

It is important to know if your ozone generator is working properly. There are two ways to know if the unit is producing ozone.

1. **Sniff for ozone**. Ozone has a distinctive smell, like the fresh smell of the air after a thunderstorm, because lightning makes ozone in nature. Just sniff; do not inhale deeply. Ozone gas can irritate the lungs and make you cough. Some portable ozone generators must warm up before producing ozone. Wait for up to one minute to do the sniff test.

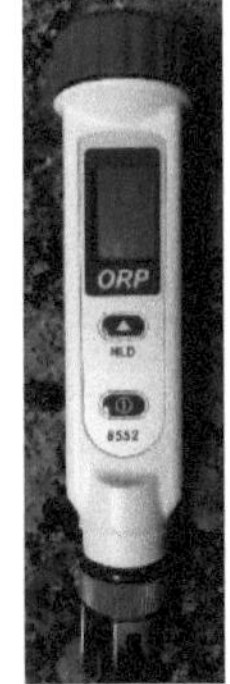

2. **Purchase an ORP meter**. Oxygen reduction potential (ORP) is the measurement of the amount of oxygen in the water. The more oxygen in the water, the more sterile it is. An ORP reading of 400 indicates water disinfection, and 600 indicates water sterilization.

Water with high ORP (400+), will disinfect or sterilize almost any surface it touches in the first twenty minutes. After that time, the water will remain disinfected and the surface will remain disinfected, but the water will no longer disinfect surfaces. [33]

Historical note: Most public water companies use ozone to disinfect their water before distribution. All bottled water companies are mandated to use ozone as a water treatment in commercial bottling.

Surfaces should be cleaned with soap before being disinfected with ozone water, because ozone water will not remove or penetrate oil.

Ozone water treatment should be used in coordination with a medical professional's recommendations. Ask your doctor if disinfecting your skin, infection, or wound with ozone water will cause any issues with healing. My experience is that most doctors have little or no knowledge of ozone water. The most common comment from doctors is, "Whatever you are doing, keep it up. You are a fast healer."

How to apply ozone water.

Ozone water is extremely powerful. It is 150% more powerful than bleach. Remember, it destroys 99.99% of bacteria and virus on contact. A small amount sprayed on the body is enough for daily skin disinfection. Ozone water should be applied more heavily to infected skin areas. It is not necessary to shower with ozone water. A small amount sprayed on the body is enough to disinfect the body.

Spray

Use a chemical-resistant pump up sprayer. These sprayers can be found in any hardware store. The best sprayer is a pump-up sprayer, because it puts pressure on the ozone water that prolongs its effectiveness, is easy to use, and has a very adjustable

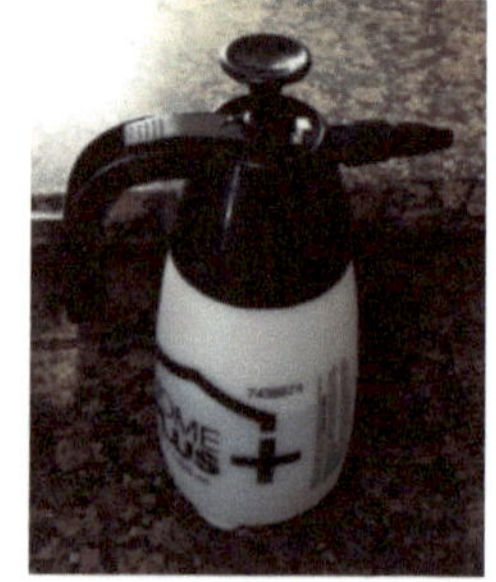

spray. Fill the sprayer ¾ full of water, and bubble for a minimum of five minutes. Replace the top, pump up, and spray.

Microfiber cloth

It is best to use a microfiber cloth, which is synthetic and antimicrobial. Soak the cloth in ozone water, then use it to wipe surfaces to disinfect. The cloth can also be used as a compress to help prevent skin infections. Be sure to rewet the cloth with ozone water every two to three minutes. Continue to bubble during compress application.

Immersion

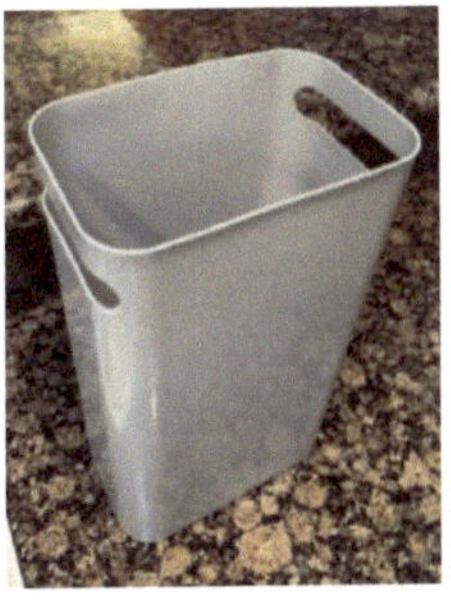

Place the body part in a properly-sized container filled with ozone water. A clean plastic bucket will work for hands, feet, and ankles. Continue to add ozone with a bubble-stone ozone generator during application. Applications should last up to thirty minutes. You can also use a bathtub or a jacuzzi to soak your entire body. Use caution to prevent your ozone generator from falling into the water. In the bath or jacuzzi, place bubble stone under the body part you want to treat. You can wear a shirt or swimsuit to trap the ozone close to your skin. Bubble for thirty minutes.

Health and Wellness

Ozone Water is the world's safest, most powerful disinfectant. You can disinfect almost any surface, including your skin, mouth, and throat. [1,2,3,4]

Bacteria and virus growth are divided into four phases:

1. Lag phase – The population of bacteria is not large enough to make you ill. This phase can last for several days before bacteria begin to 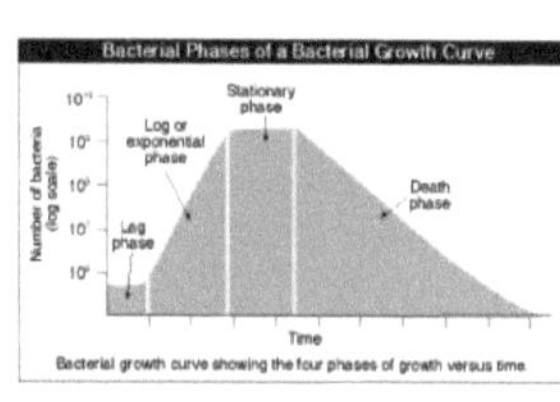

   multiply and move to the next stage.
2. Log, or exponential phase – As the number of bacteria multiply exponentially, they produce toxins. When enough toxins are produced, you begin to feel ill.
3. Stationary phase – High bacterial count produces high levels of toxins and makes you feel ill.
4. Death phase – Bacteria die off, the toxins are reduced, and you begin to feel better. You may now have secondary infections that must be treated before you are completely well.

We live in a world filled with numerous bacteria. Bacteria can never be eliminated, but they can be controlled by daily applications of ozone water.

In the lag phase, there is not a large enough population of bacteria or viruses to make you ill. You begin to feel the illness in the log phase as the bacteria find a host tissue and experience exponential growth. Ozone water disinfection keeps bacterial or viral cells in the lag phase by destroying and controlling the growth of the pathogen population before they can enter the exponential growth phase. You are prevented from becoming ill because the pathogen cannot expand its population to the point of illness requiring medical attention. A vast majority of bacteria and viruses enter the body via the mouth, nose, and throat. These bacteria require several days to reach the log phase. Gargling with ozone water daily will destroy most of these bacteria daily. This prevents population of bacteria from reaching the second phase of growth and prevents you from feeling ill.

Ozone water will not prevent every illness, because pathogens have numerous ways to enter the body. However, if you do become ill, gargling with ozone water will lessen the severity of the illness by preventing sore throat and oral infections. Gargling with ozone water will also help prevent the spread of a disease to people that you encounter. [1,15]

Historical note: *During WWI, ozone was used to treat wounds, trench foot, gangrene, and the effects of poison gas. *(4)*

Ozone water also promotes rapid healing by providing oxygen to the skin. It has been known since the 1850s that oxygen is absorbed by the skin. When you spray or immerse your skin in ozone water, the high concentration of activated oxygen diffuses through the skin, and is then absorbed by the blood and transported by the circulatory system to the site of the injury. Oxygen is the most important ingredient for healing. Remember: **more oxygen = less infection = faster healing**. [10,11,12,16,17,19]

Historical note: Swiss dentist E.A. Fisch was using ozone in dentistry before 1932, and introduced it to German surgeon Erwin Payr, who used it from that time forward. [4]

Less infection will reduce the need for antibiotics. The reduction of antibiotic use has been recommended for years, but never advanced. Reduced antibiotic use will save money, too.

Healing involves four steps:

1. Hemostasis
2. Inflammation
3. Proliferation
4. Remodeling

Ozone water will prevent inflammation and shorten or eliminate the inflammation stage of healing. Prevention of inflammation will speed healing by 20-30%, and has the added benefit of reduced scarring. [11, 16]

How to use ozone water to help promote good health and wellness

a. **Help prevent cold and flu**

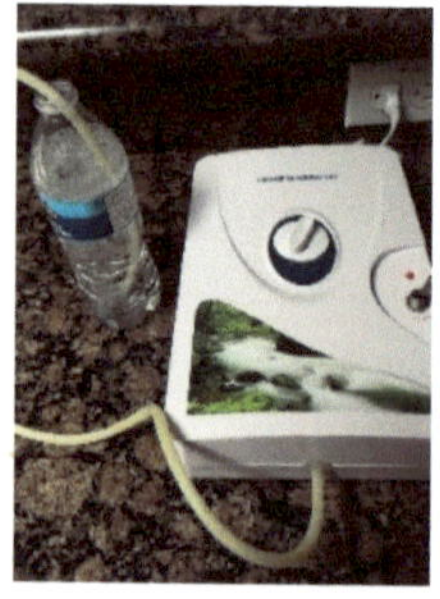

– The average American has two to three cold/flu events per year. Ozone water will reduce this by 50% or more. Gargle with ozone water several times per day to disinfect mouth and throat. Most pathogens enter the body via the mouth, nose and throat. Gargling with ozone water daily will destroy pathogens before they can multiply and make you sick. If you do get sick, gargling with ozone water will reduce the severity of the disease by preventing sore throat and oral infections. Bubble ozone into a water bottle or glass for a minimum of five minutes. Gargle and rinse mouth. It is safe to swallow the ozone water. [15]

b. **Help promote rapid healing of skin**

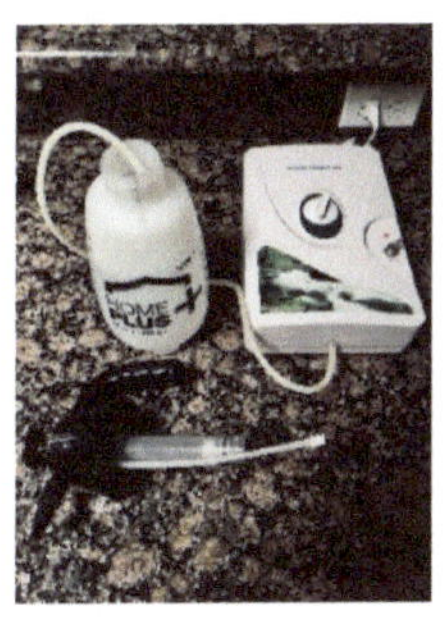

– Spray ozone water on clean skin wounds and infections once or twice per day. A daily ozone water spray to the skin will prevent most skin infections. The ozone spray destroys virus, bacteria, and mold on the skin. The easiest way to do this is by disinfecting your body during a shower. [10,11,12,16,17,18,19]

c. **Disinfect body during shower**

– After shampoo and soap are applied and rinsed, use the sprayer to spray your entire body with ozone water. It is not necessary to stop your shower water, so you can stay warm and comfortable while spraying. Remove a body part from the water stream and spray with ozone water. Continue to spray from top down until entire body has been disinfected. Activated oxygen is absorbed faster when the skin is damp. Use additional spray on infections, bruises, or wounds. Adjust to fine spray for mouth, and inhale fine mist of ozone water to disinfect mouth, throat, and nose. Be sure to rinse your navel. Disinfecting your body daily will eliminate body odor and promote good health and wellness organically. Spray the remaining ozone water on the walls of the shower to freshen the shower and prevent mold and mildew. Ozone water will also help clean the drain of biofilm.

Historical note: In a 2012 study published by PLOS One, researchers found 2,368 species of bacteria nestled into the navel, 1,485 of which may be new to science. Ozone water will destroy 99.99% of all bacteria on contact.

d. **Help promote healing of non-healing wounds.**

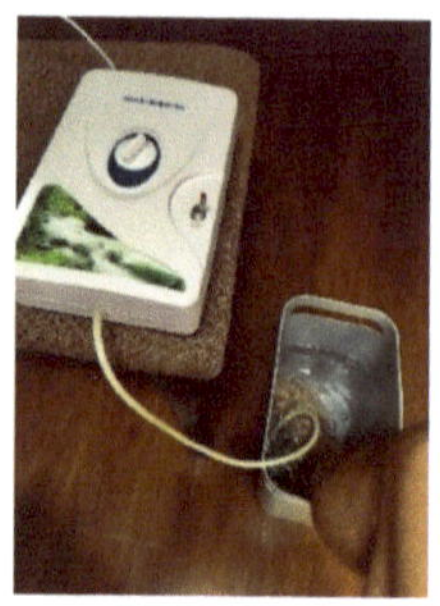

Ozone water destroys the bacterial biofilm that is present in non-healing wounds. Wounds on hands and feet can be immersed in a container of water that has been ozonized. Use bubble stone to continue adding ozone to the water while immersing for thirty minutes, allowing bubbles to flow over the affected area. For larger body parts, apply spray during shower, following shower spray directions. Another option is to soak a microfiber cloth in ozone water and apply as a compress over the affected area. Continue to bubble ozone into water container, rewet cloth every several minutes, and reapply to wound. Treat wound several times per day for ten to fifteen minutes. [15,16]

e. **Help promote rapid healing of burns and sunburn.**

Ozone water will promote rapid healing of burns by disinfection and oxygenation of the burn. It is best to use RO water on burns for two reasons: the ozone content in RO water will be higher than tap water, and purer water will leave little to no dissolved solids on the burn. Begin ozone water application as soon as possible after the burn happens. Spray or immerse the burn with ozone water once or twice per day to help prevent infection and promote rapid healing. Allow the burn to air-dry.

NOTE: For severe burns, get immediate medical attention.

f. **Help prevent acne, diaper rash, bed sores, and other skin infections.**

Daily application of ozone water will help prevent skin infections—even flesh-eating bacteria are destroyed by ozone water. Be sure to clean skin with soap before applying ozone water. Apply ozone water to skin infection via spray or microfiber cloth once or twice daily.

g. **Help promote healthy teeth and gums.**

Ozone water will kill bacteria that cause plaque and oral diseases while promoting healthy teeth and gums. Rinse mouth with ozone water after brushing and flossing.

h. **Help promote healing after dental procedures.**

Gargling with ozone water after a dental procedure will disinfect your mouth and help prevent infection and promote rapid healing.

i. **Eliminate bad breath.**

Ozone water will destroy the bacteria that cause bad breath. Rinse mouth with ozone water several times per day as needed.

j. **Help promote rapid healing of insect and spider bites.**

Ozone water helps neutralize spider venom, just as it does other organic material. Spray, soak, or use microfiber cloth to apply ozone water to affected area. Repeat as necessary, at least twice per day to promote rapid healing of the bite. Note: Seek medical attention immediately if severe pain, redness, or swelling persist.

Food Safety

The Food and Drug Administration (FDA) has approved the use of ozone water for food safety to prevent foodborne illnesses. Ozone water destroys 99.99% of virus and bacteria on contact, and will disinfect almost any surface, including fruits and vegetables. The FDA has approved ozone water for use as a food additive, and for disinfection of food, food contact surfaces, and surfaces in general. [6, 21,22]

Historical note: The U.S. Food and Drug Administration formally approved the use of ozone as an antimicrobial agent for the treatment, storage, and processing of foods in gas and aqueous phases. The approval was published on June 26, 2001.

Romaine lettuce has been known to cause foodborne illnesses if not properly disinfected. Ozone water is the easiest and best method to disinfect lettuce, enhancing flavor and leaving no chemical residue. Chemical vegetable disinfectants require longer treatment time, and leave a residue that affects flavor and digestion of the lettuce.

How to use ozone water in food safety

a. **Disinfect food contact surfaces.**

– Clean utensils, cutting boards, and serving plates with ozone water. Wipe countertops and surfaces with damp microfiber cloth, or spray with ozone water and wipe dry.

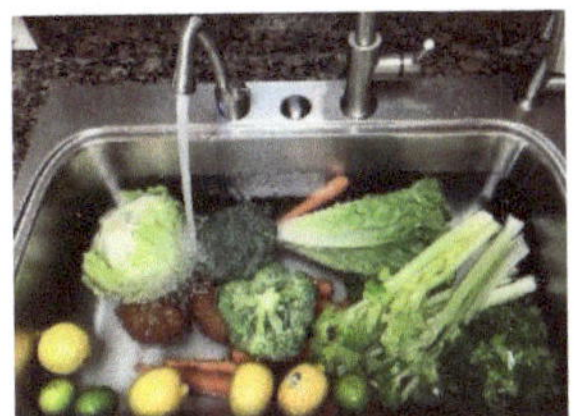

b. **Disinfect fruits and vegetables to extend storage life.**

— Place fruits and vegetables into vessel of ozone water. Continue to add ozone with bubble stone unit. Allow produce to sit for several minutes in the ozone water. Drain, dry, and 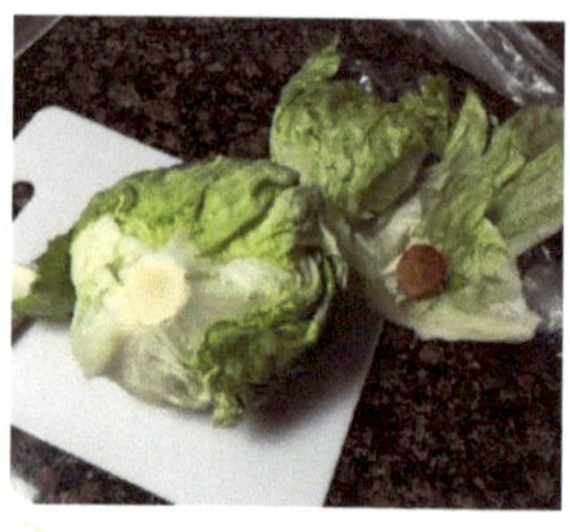 place in open plastic bag with paper towel. Do not seal bag. Ozone water disinfection can double the storage life of fruits and vegetables.

c. **Disinfect romaine and head lettuce.**

— Ozone water revives lettuce from limp to loud. Lettuce that has been soaked in ozone water and chilled will attain maximum crispness. For 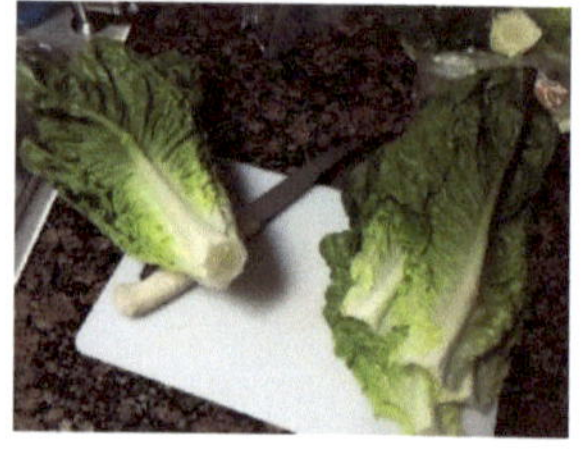 immediate use, remove the stalk and separate the leaves. Soak leaves in ozone water for several minutes, drain, and refrigerate. For long-term storage, cut a small slice off the stalk to expose fresh stalk, and remove outer leaves. Soak lettuce in ozone water for two to five minutes; drain well. Place lettuce head in plastic bag along with a paper towel (do not seal bag), and refrigerate. This method also works well for broccoli, celery, and other vegetables with stalks.

d. **Remove pesticides.**

– Soak fruits and vegetables in ozone water for several minutes to remove pesticides. Pesticides are destroyed by ozone water. ***Take the strawberry taste test:*** rinse several strawberries in tap water and several strawberries in ozone water. Take a bite of the ozone-treated berry, then take a bite of the other one. You can taste the difference.

e. **Improve flavor of fish and poultry.**

– Fish and poultry can develop a bacterial biofilm coating that causes odors and adversely affects taste. Ozone water destroys this biofilm as well as the odors. Rinse or spray fish and poultry with ozone water to remove the biofilm and improve flavor. Rinse fish and poultry once before freezing, and again before cooking for maximum flavor.

f. **Improve flavor and quality of drinking water.**

– For the best-tasting water, do what every water bottler is required to do. Bubble ozone water for a minimum of five minutes, then allow water to sit for twenty minutes to remove ozone odor. Refrigerate the water, if desired. Ozone water will also disinfect the container holding it. This makes it a safe and flavorful method for refilling water bottles.

g. **Improve flavor of beverages.**

– Coffee, tea, lemonade, and other beverages will taste better if ozone water is used to make them. Ozone water will remove any unwanted odors or flavors, leaving you with great-tasting beverages.

h. **Extend storage life of grains.**

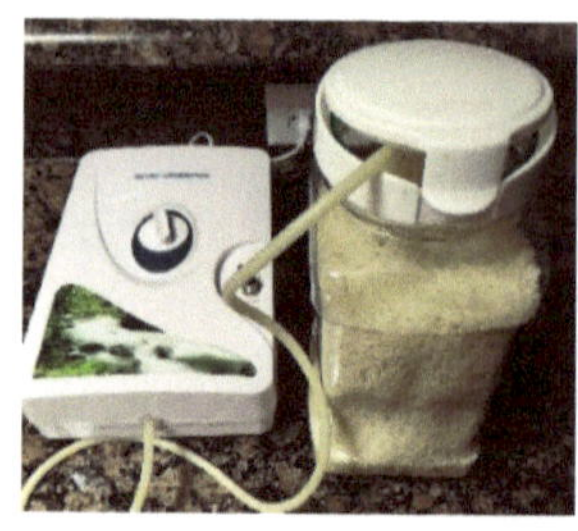

– Ozone gas will destroy the eggs and larva of any insects in the grain. Place bubble stone at bottom of grain container and cover, allowing air to escape. Apply ozone gas for thirty minutes. Seal the container. The ozone gas will disinfect the grain and destroy any insect eggs or larva. Sealing the container immediately after treatment will prolong storage life.

i. **Clean drains.**

– Ozone water destroys bacterial biofilm in drains. This helps keep the drain clean. The ozone water will also prevent fruit flies and other sewer-dwelling insects, by destroying the biofilm they consume and destroying their eggs and larva.

j. **Eliminate cooking odors.**

– Run the ozone generator into the air while cooking. Ozone gas will eliminate the odors. ***Take the garlic test.*** Rub a garlic clove into the palm of your hand. Smell hand. Rinse hand with ozone water. Smell again; the garlic odor is gone. Under normal circumstances, the garlic smell would take several days to go away. No amount of soap and water will eliminate the odor as quickly.

Athletic Applications for Ozone Water

Ozone water immersion (OWI) can promote rapid healing of athletic injuries, prevent skin infections, and reduce the inflammation that slows performances. Earlier chapters described how ozone water promotes rapid healing. OWI will also help promote rapid healing of bruises and sprains, and reduce inflammation. OWI simply involves putting your hand, foot, or body into a container of ozone water, and "bubble" by continuing to add ozone for thirty minutes. As the ozone becomes activated oxygen, it is absorbed by the skin, picked up by the blood, and transported to the site of the injury. Continue to add ozone to the container while bubbling to keep the ozone content as high as possible. It is best to begin immersion therapy as soon as possible after the injury.

How to use ozone water in athletics

a. **Disinfect showers, training tables, and mats.**

– Use warm, soapy water to remove any grease, oil, or film from surface. Apply ozone water to surfaces that need disinfection via spray or microfiber cloth. Wipe dry with microfiber cloth, or let air dry. Ozone water will prevent mold and mildew, disinfect surfaces, eliminate odors, and destroy MRSA virus. [1,3,4,12]

b. **Athlete's foot, jock itch, and other bacterial, viral and fungal skin infections.**

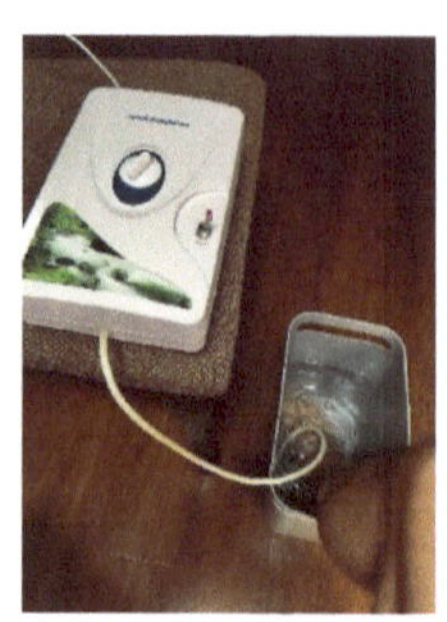

– Use ozone water immersion. Soak athlete's foot in ozone water for thirty minutes per day, or spray ozone water on entire body while in shower. Apply extra spray to affected areas.

c. **Sprains.**

– Use ozone water immersion. Soak hand or foot and ankle in ozone water for thirty minutes, several times per day. Continue to bubble water while applying. Begin application as soon as possible after injury.

d. **Bruises.**

– Use ozone water immersion. Soak, spray, or use microfiber cloth compress on bruise with ozone water. A strong spray applied directly to the bruise will visibly reduce it during application. Begin application as soon as possible after injury. Bubble for thirty minutes.

e. **Reduce inflammation.**

– Ozone water immersion will provide activated oxygen, which is absorbed by the skin and transported to the site of inflammation by the blood to reduce inflammation. Oxygen is the most important component of healing, and ozone water delivers large quantities of it to the site of injury. Bubble for thirty minutes. [13]

f. **Eliminate equipment odors.**

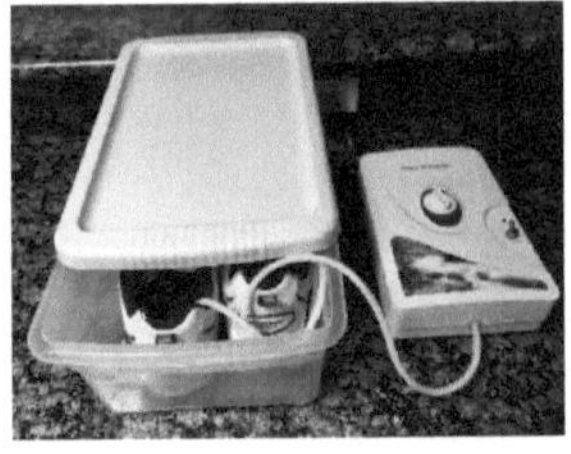

– Clean equipment first, then place helmets, pads, shoes, and other equipment into a plastic bag or container. Pump ozone gas into container for ten to twenty minutes. Allow some air to escape from bag, but keep bag closed. After ten to twenty minutes, seal bag with equipment until next use.

Veterinary

Ozone water is the world's safest, most powerful disinfectant. You can disinfect almost any surface, including your pet's skin. Ozone water will promote good health and wellness in your pets, just as it does for humans, because oxygen diffuses through animal skin, too. It will soothe and disinfect skin irritations from hot spots, fleas, ticks, and other skin irritants. [24,25,26,27,28]

HOW TO USE OZONE WATER TO PROMOTE GOOD HEALTH AND WELLNESS FOR YOUR PETS

   a. **Help prevent skin infection.**

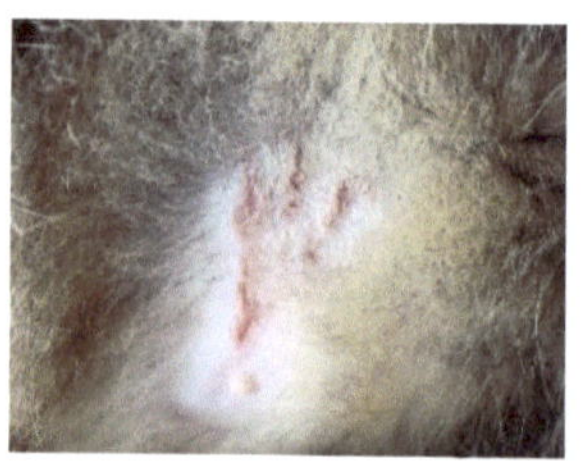

   – Apply ozone water with spray or microfiber cloth, or bathe pet in ozone water. Continue to bubble ozone into water during bath. Cats prefer to be wiped down with a damp microfiber cloth. Dry pets after treatment. Ozone water will promote rapid healing by preventing infection. Photo shows a cat scratch healing without infection or antibiotics.

   b. **Help prevent post-surgery infections.**

   – Follow veterinarian's directions. Apply ozone water with spray, bath, or microfiber cloth as soon as possible to promote rapid healing. Repeat several times per day, as necessary.

c. **Flea and tick prevention.**

– Ozone water kills the eggs and larva of skin-dwelling insects. Ozone water will not kill adult insects. Bathe pets in ozone water frequently to prevent young insects from hatching.

d. **How to bathe your pet:**

   i. **Dogs**. Prepare ozone water for rinsing in advance of bath, and continue to bubble. Place dog in tub large enough to hold the animal and the ozone water. Shampoo and rinse with ozone water, using a microfiber cloth. Dry with a clean, dry towel. Give the dog a treat and praise after the bath to encourage him/her to do it again.

   ii. **Cats**: Place cat on counter top or other smooth hard surface where it can't get traction. Gently hold the cat with one hand and speak softly to keep him/her calm. Soak microfiber cloth in ozone water. Gently rub cat's fur back and forth with the moist cloth so ozone water can reach the cat's skin. Dry with clean, dry cloth. Give the cat a treat and praise to encourage him/her to do it again.

e. **Help promote healthy teeth and gums**

– and prevent infection after oral surgery. Spray ozone water into pet's mouth. Many animals prefer the flavor of ozone water to regular water. Fill bowl with ozone water and encourage pet to drink.

e. **Help prevent bad breath in pets.**

– Spray mouth with ozone water, or allow pet to drink fresh ozone water daily.

f. **Eliminate pet odors.**

– Ozone water eliminates odors by destroying the bacteria that cause odors. Flush kennels with ozone water after cleaning. Bathe pets in ozone water to eliminate the bacteria on their skin that causes odors. Have pets drink ozone water to freshen their breath. Ozone water also disinfects stinky ears and soothes hot spots.

Plants

Ozone water is the safest, most powerful disinfectant available. You can disinfect almost any surface, including your plants. Ozone water is approved by the EPA for use as an organic pesticide, and destroys mold and mildew. [7,28,29]

a. **Extend the life of cut flowers.**

– Cut one inch off stalks of new flowers. Place flowers in ozone water and bubble for thirty minutes. Replace water, and bubble with ozone as needed.

b. **Organic pesticide.**

Ozone water is an EPA-approved organic pesticide. Spray plants completely, from the top and bottom of leaves to the stalks. Ozone water destroys the eggs and larva of insects; however, it will not affect adult insects.

c. **Promote healthy clones.**

Clip clones from the mother plant, then dip into ozone water to promote mold-free growth and uptake of nutrient solution.

d. **Promote nutrient uptake of fertilizer.**

Apply fertilizer following directions, then water the plant with ozone water. Ozone water breaks fertilizer's nitrogen into nitrates that are easily absorbed by the plant, which increases flower and fruit production.

e. **Eliminate mold.**

Ozone water destroys mold. Mist plants daily with ozone water for prevention.

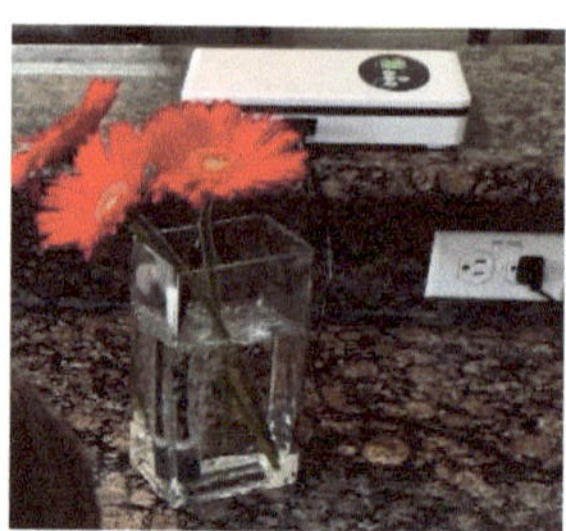 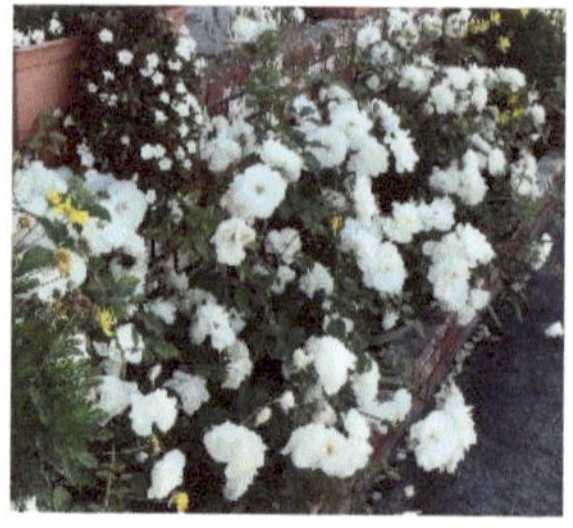

Conclusion

Education is vital to the acceptance of ozone water. Ozone water is not well understood, because it is contrary to everything we have been told about disinfection.

- "Hot water and soap kill bacteria."
- "Don't get your wound wet; it will get infected."
- "Disinfectants must have a chemical smell, like chlorine."

Every American, at one time or another, will have a problem with bacteria, viruses, or other pathogens. Why not use ozone water?

- Government-approved for disinfection.
- Destroys 99.99% of viruses and bacteria on contact.
- Ozone water will help prevent and reduce the severity of cold/flu.
- Ozone water will help prevent skin infections.
- 100% organic. Contains only activated oxygen and water.
- Has been called "the world's safest therapy."
- Inexpensive.
- Easy to produce.
- Very effective.

We live with a daily struggle against bacteria and viruses. Many strains of bacteria are becoming more and more resistant to antibiotics. However, they cannot become resistant to ozone water. Ozone water will give you the upper hand in this struggle. You will now have "Superman" on your side.

Ozone water is the world's safest, most powerful disinfectant, yet most people have never heard of it. Why is this? Why does the term "ozone" strike fear in so many people? I believe the answer to these questions is best summed up by Saul Pressman in *The Story of Ozone*, in which he states, "In 1933, the American Medical Association, headed by Dr. Simmons, set out to destroy all medical treatments that were competitive to drug therapy. The suppression of ozone therapy continues in the U.S. to this day."

Ozone water has the ability to drastically reduce the use of antibiotics. This reduction of antibiotics has been promoted for years, but not implemented. [4]

Ozone water delivers many benefits that promote good health and wellness in people, pets, and plants, organically and at low cost. A portable ozone generator costs less than $100.00. On-demand ozone faucets cost between $600 and $1,200, plus installation. This is a small price to pay to reduce your chance of illness and help promote rapid healing. The best option is to purchase an ozone faucet for the convenience of ozone on demand, and a portable ozone generator for bubbling applications and travel.

OzoneForYou.com offers portable ozone generators and ozone faucets for sale. Order your units today, and sign up for the newsletter to begin using ozone water to promote good health and wellness for people, pets, and plants. Please comment on our Facebook page about your experience with ozone water.

End Notes

GENERAL OZONE KNOWLEDGE

(1) Lillard, Susan. 2004. "How Ozone Affects Bacteria, Fungus, Molds and Viruses." https://sportsozone.com/index.php/download_file/view/49/161/.

(2) Franken, Laurence. 2001. "The Application of Ozone Technology for Public Health and Industry." *Population.* http://emo3.com/wp-content/uploads/2015/07/White-Paper-Kansas-State-University.pdf.

(3) Adachi, Ken. 2002. "Ozone, A Quick Overview." 2002. http://educate-yourself.org/ozone/.

(4) Pressman, Saul, and Otto Heinrich Warburg. 2000. *The Story of Ozone.* Accessed September 29, 2018. http://uralica.com/oz.htm.

(5) Friedman, Daniel. n.d. "Ozone Gas Exposure Standards: Ozone Gas Hazards, Ozone Generators: Standards for Using Ozone Treatments for Mold in Buildings." Accessed September 29, 2018. https://www.inspectapedia.com/sickhouse/Ozone_Exposure_Standards.php.

GOVERNMENTAL APPROVAL

(6) "Science & Research (Food) - Chapter V. Methods to Reduce/Eliminate Pathogens from Produce and Fresh-Cut Produce." 2014. US Food and Drug Administration. https://www.fda.gov/Food/FoodScienceResearch/ucm091363.htm.

(7) "Water Treatability Database." 2007. US Environmental Protection Agency. https://iaspub.epa.gov/tdb/pages/treatment/treatmentOverview.do?treatmentProcessId=-1467636837.

(8) EPA pesticide approval, https://OzoneForYou.com/ozone-resources

(9) USDA/ National Organic Program (NOP). n.d. "SDA National Organic Program Ozone Approval." http://www.tersano.com/.

PEOPLE

(10) Sen, Chandan K. 2009. "Wound Healing Essentials: Let There Be Oxygen." *Wound Repair and Regeneration: Official Publication of the Wound Healing Society [and] the European Tissue Repair Society* 17 (1): 1–18.

(11) Guo, S., and L. A. Dipietro. 2010. "Factors Affecting Wound Healing." *Journal of Dental Research* 89 (3): 219–29.

(12) Sunnen, G. 1998. "The Utilization of Ozone for External Medical Applications." *Journal of Advanced Medical-Surgical Nursing* 1: 159–74.

(13) Azuma, Kazuo, Takuro Mori, Kinya Kawamoto, Kohei Kuroda, Takeshi Tsuka, Tomohiro Imagawa, Tomohiro Osaki, Fumio Itoh, Saburo Minami, and Yoshiharu Okamoto. 2014. "Anti-Inflammatory Effects of Ozonated Water in an Experimental Mouse Model." *Biomedical Reports* 2 (5): 671–74.

(14) Sadatullah, Syed. 2013. "Ozonated Water an Adjunct to Tooth Brushing and Flossing. Myth or Reality?" In *Microbial Pathogens and Strategies for Combating Them: Science, Technology and Education*, edited by A. Méndez-Vilas. Formatex Research Center.

(15) Connor, Erinn. 2018. "Cold and Flu 101: What You Need to Know | Everyday Health." EverydayHealth.com. August 28, 2018.
https://www.everydayhealth.com/flu/guide/.

SKIN

(16) Biology of Wound Healing, what goes wrong when wounds don't heal:
https://www.fda.gov/downloads/AdvisoryCommittees/CommitteesMeetingMaterials/MedicalDevices/MedicalDevicesAdvisoryCommittee/GeneralandPlasticSurgeryDevicesPanel/UCM522886.pdf

(17) Bialoszewski, Dariusz, Anna Pietruczuk-Padzik, Agnieszka Kalicinska, Ewa Bocian, Magdalena Czajkowska, Bozena Bukowska, and Stefan Tyski. 2011. "Activity of Ozonated Water and Ozone against Staphylococcus Aureus and Pseudomonas Aeruginosa Biofilms." *Medical Science Monitor: International Medical Journal of Experimental and Clinical Research* 17 (11): BR339–44.

(18) Stücker, M., A. Struk, P. Altmeyer, M. Herde, H. Baumgärtl, and D. W. Lübbers. 2002. "The Cutaneous Uptake of Atmospheric Oxygen Contributes Significantly to the Oxygen Supply of Human Dermis and Epidermis." *The Journal of Physiology* 538 (Pt 3): 985–94.

(19) The National Academies. n.d. "How Infection Works, Entering the Human Host." What You Need To Know About Infectious Disease. Accessed September 29, 2018.
http://needtoknow.nas.edu/id/infection/encountering-microbes/entering-the-human-host/.

(20) Soodak, H., and A. Iberall. 1978. "Osmosis, Diffusion, Convection." *The American Journal of Physiology* 235 (1): R3–17.

FOOD SAFETY

(21) Hinkle, Bruce. 2017. "Ozone as an Added Protection in Food Processing Chain - Food Quality & Safety." Food Quality & Safety. July 20, 2017. http://www.foodqualityandsafety.com/article/ozone-added-protection-food-processing-chain/.

(22) Donnelly, Laura. 2017.. "Organic Foods Backed by Landmark Report Warning Pesticides Far More Dangerous than Was Thought." *The Daily Telegraph*, June 2, 2017. https://www.telegraph.co.uk/news/2017/06/02/organic-foods-backed-landmark-report-warning-pesticides-far/

(23) Brandt, Jim. 2008. "Ozone Re-Emerges as an Economical and Green Safety Tool - Food Quality & Safety." Food Quality & Safety. December 1, 2008. http://www.foodqualityandsafety.com/article/the-case-for-ozone/.

PETS

(24) skeptvet. n.d. "Ozone Therapy for Pets | The SkeptVet." Accessed September 29, 2018. http://skeptvet.com/Blog/2012/08/ozone-therapy-for-pets/.

(24) "Veterinary Holistic Care: Ozone Therapy." n.d. Accessed September 29, 2018. http://www.vhcdoc.com/resources/OzoneTheraphy.html.

(26) Roman, Margo, DVM, CVA, COT, and CPT. 2013. "Ozone Therapy in the Veterinary Practice - IVC Journal." IVC Journal. September 12, 2013. http://ivcjournal.com/ozone-therapy-in-the-veterinary-practice/.

(27) Newkirk, Mark. 2014. "Ozone Therapy for Animals." *Animal Wellness Magazine*, March 11, 2014. https://animalwellnessmagazine.com/ozone-therapy/.

(28) Ptashkin, Samantha. 2016. "Ozone Treatment Saves Abandoned Dog's Life." *KPRC*. http://www.click2houston.com/news/ozone-treatment-saves-abadoned-dogs-life.

PLANTS

(29) Wasteland, Baron. 2014. "Ozone: An Indoor Garden Super Tool." *Maximum Yield*, February 18, 2014. https://www.maximumyield.com/ozone-an-indoor-garden-super-tool/2/1165.

(30) Rich, Ted, and Ed Knueve. 2002. "[PDF]A Look at Ozone in Hydroponics Applications - Ozomax." *Water Technology Magazine*, September 2002. http://www.ozomax.com/pdf/hydroponics.pdf.

SUPPRESSION OF OZONE:

(31) skeptvet. n.d. "Ozone Therapy for Pets | The SkeptVet." Accessed September 29, 2018. http://skeptvet.com/Blog/2012/08/ozone-therapy-for-pets/.

HOW OZONE WORKS

(32) Leusink, Joel. 2010. "How Does Ozone Kill Bacteria?" Ozone Journal. March 28, 2010. https://www.ozonesolutions.com/journal/2010/how-does-ozone-kill-bacteria/.

ORP

(33) Rappaport, Tina. 2005. "What Is ORP - Oxidation Reduction Potential." May 18, 2005. http://urparamount.com/articles/ORP/what-orp.html.

Fact Check

Adachi, Ken. 2002. "Ozone, A Quick Overview." http://educate-yourself.org/ozone/.

Azuma, Kazuo, Takuro Mori, Kinya Kawamoto, Kohei Kuroda, Takeshi Tsuka, Tomohiro Imagawa, Tomohiro Osaki, Fumio Itoh, Saburo Minami, and Yoshiharu Okamoto. 2014. "Anti-Inflammatory Effects of Ozonated Water in an Experimental Mouse Model." *Biomedical Reports* 2 (5): 671–74.

Bialoszewski, Dariusz, Anna Pietruczuk-Padzik, Agnieszka Kalicinska, Ewa Bocian, Magdalena Czajkowska, Bozena Bukowska, and Stefan Tyski. 2011. "Activity of Ozonated Water and Ozone against Staphylococcus Aureus and Pseudomonas Aeruginosa Biofilms." *Medical Science Monitor: International Medical Journal of Experimental and Clinical Research* 17 (11): BR339–44.

Brandt, Jim. 2008. "Ozone Re-Emerges as an Economical and Green Safety Tool - Food Quality & Safety." Food Quality & Safety. December 1, 2008. http://www.foodqualityandsafety.com/article/the-case-for-ozone/.

Connor, Erinn. 2018. "Cold and Flu 101: What You Need to Know | Everyday Health." EverydayHealth.com. August 28, 2018. https://www.everydayhealth.com/flu/guide/.

Donnelly, Laura. 2017. "Organic Foods Backed by Landmark Report Warning Pesticides Far More Dangerous than Was Thought." *The Daily Telegraph*, June 2, 2017. https://www.telegraph.co.uk/news/2017/06/02/organic-foods-backed-landmark-report-warning-pesticides-far/.

Franken, Laurence. 2001. "The Application of Ozone Technology for Public Health and Industry." *Population.* http://emo3.com/wp-content/uploads/2015/07/White-Paper-Kansas-State-University.pdf.

Friedman, Daniel. n.d. "Ozone Gas Exposure Standards: Ozone Gas Hazards, Ozone Generators: Standards for Using Ozone Treatments for Mold in Buildings." Accessed September 29, 2018. https://www.inspectapedia.com/sickhouse/Ozone_Exposure_Standards.php.

Guo, S., and L. A. Dipietro. 2010. "Factors Affecting Wound Healing." *Journal of Dental Research* 89 (3): 219–29.

Hinkle, Bruce. 2017. "Ozone as an Added Protection in Food Processing Chain - Food Quality & Safety." Food Quality & Safety. July 20, 2017. http://www.foodqualityandsafety.com/article/ozone-added-protection-food-processing-chain/.

Leusink, Joel. 2010. "How Does Ozone Kill Bacteria?" Ozone Journal. March 28, 2010. https://www.ozonesolutions.com/journal/2010/how-does-ozone-kill-bacteria/.

Lillard, Susan. 2004. "How Ozone Affects Bacteria, Fungus, Molds and Viruses." https://sportsozone.com/index.php/download_file/view/49/161/.

The National Academies. n.d. "How Infection Works, Entering the Human Host." What You Need To Know About Infectious Disease. Accessed September 29, 2018. http://needtoknow.nas.edu/id/infection/encountering-microbes/entering-the-human-host/.

Newkirk, Mark. 2014. "Ozone Therapy for Animals." *Animal Wellness Magazine*, March 11, 2014. https://animalwellnessmagazine.com/ozone-therapy/.

Pressman, Saul, and Otto Heinrich Warburg. 2000. *The Story of Ozone.* Accessed September 29, 2018. http://uralica.com/oz.htm.

Ptashkin, Samantha. 2016. "Ozone Treatment Saves Abandoned Dog's Life." *KPRC.* http://www.click2houston.com/news/ozone-treatment-saves-abadoned-dogs-life.

Rappaport, Tina. 2005. "What Is ORP - Oxidation Reduction Potential." May 18, 2005. http://urparamount.com/articles/ORP/what-orp.html.

Rich, Ted, and Ed Knueve. 2002. "[PDF]A Look at Ozone in Hydroponics Applications - Ozomax." *Water Technology Magazine*, September 2002. http://www.ozomax.com/pdf/hydroponics.pdf.

Roman, Margo, DVM, CVA, COT, and CPT. 2013. "Ozone Therapy in the Veterinary Practice - IVC Journal." IVC Journal. September 12, 2013. http://ivcjournal.com/ozone-therapy-in-the-veterinary-practice/.

Sadatullah, Syed. 2013. "Ozonated Water an Adjunct to Tooth Brushing and Flossing. Myth or Reality?" In *Microbial Pathogens and Strategies for Combating Them: Science, Technology and Education*, edited by A. Méndez-Vilas. Formatex Research Center.

"Science & Research (Food) - Chapter V. Methods to Reduce/Eliminate Pathogens from Produce and Fresh-Cut Produce." 2014. US Food and Drug Administration. https://www.fda.gov/Food/FoodScienceResearch/ucm091363.htm.

Sen, Chandan K. 2009. "Wound Healing Essentials: Let There Be Oxygen." *Wound Repair and Regeneration: Official Publication of the Wound Healing Society [and] the European Tissue Repair Society* 17 (1): 1–18.

Skeptvet. n.d. "Ozone Therapy for Pets | The SkeptVet." Accessed September 29, 2018. http://skeptvet.com/Blog/2012/08/ozone-therapy-for-pets/.

Soodak, H., and A. Iberall. 1978. "Osmosis, Diffusion, Convection." *The American Journal of Physiology* 235 (1): R3–17.

Stücker, M., A. Struk, P. Altmeyer, M. Herde, H. Baumgärtl, and D. W. Lübbers. 2002. "The Cutaneous Uptake of Atmospheric Oxygen Contributes Significantly to the Oxygen Supply of Human Dermis and Epidermis." *The Journal of Physiology* 538 (Pt 3): 985–94.

Sunnen, G. 1998. "The Utilization of Ozone for External Medical Applications." *Journal of Advanced Medical-Surgical Nursing* 1: 159–74.

USDA/ National Organic Program (NOP). n.d. "SDA National Organic Program Ozone Approval." http://www.tersano.com/.

"Veterinary Holistic Care: Ozone Therapy." n.d. Accessed September 29, 2018. http://www.vhcdoc.com/resources/OzoneTheraphy.html.

Wasteland, Baron. 2014. "Ozone: An Indoor Garden Super Tool." *Maximum Yield*, February 18, 2014. https://www.maximumyield.com/ozone-an-indoor-garden-super-tool/2/1165.

"Water Treatability Database." 2007. US Environmental Protection Agency. https://iaspub.epa.gov/tdb/pages/treatment/treatmentOverview.do?treatmentProcessId=-1467636837.

Biography

Mike Casey, Ozone for You

I have been intimately involved with water my entire life. Water was very important to my childhood development. I began swimming competitively at the age of nine, because my family doctor recommended it to treat my asthma. I continued to swim throughout high school and swam for the University of Michigan, where I was All-American and qualified for the Olympic trials. I still swim for exercise.

The ability of swimming to cure my asthma affected my choice of study at the U of M. I majored in kinesiology, and wanted to become a physical trainer to help other athletes overcome medical issues. After teaching science at a junior high school and coaching for two years, I joined the family soft water company.

My father began a soft water business in 1954. He was awarded the Pioneer of Water Quality award by the Water Quality Association for his work in low-pressure reverse-osmosis systems. As the second son, I had to prove myself by developing new ways to sell water. I developed a pure-water division that consisted of commercial reverse osmosis and deionized water sales and service. My customers included the Jean Prison, Primm Resorts, Nellis AFB, and local hospitals. I also developed a mobile wash that serviced every new-car dealer in the region and large local trucking firms, including UPS and Silver State Disposal, the local trash company.

I left the family water business in 1978 to work at Xerox until 1985, when I purchased Lamb Asphalt Maintenance, a local pavement maintenance company. I operated Lamb Asphalt until

I sold the company in 2010 and retired to Huntington Beach.

I was introduced to Ozone Water by Bruce Hinkle, Chief Technical Officer at PureQuest Ozone Technology and one of the few experts in the field. This unknown form of water completely amazed me, and I began to experiment with it. My cat, Fred, has an allergy to human dander. He would lick himself raw. The sores would become infected and require medical attention along with antibiotics and steroids. I began to give Fred a daily wipe-down with ozone water on a microfiber cloth. Fred's sores no longer became infected. He will still lick himself raw occasionally, but the sores will heal without infection or antibiotics.

The success treating Fred with ozone water led me to begin applying ozone water to my own skin. Years of swimming outdoors in the desert had left my skin dry and prone to bruising and bleeding. Ozone water has helped this skin issue greatly. My sunspots have also been noticeably reduced.

Once, while I was out of town, my wife rolled her ankle. The injury left her alone and unable to walk, with a swollen ankle and a large bruise. Out of desperation to help her, I suggested that she soak her ankle in ozone water for thirty minutes. Amazingly, after the thirty-minute application, she was able to walk without any discomfort. She repeated the application the next morning.   After the second application, she was astonished that there was no pain, swelling, or bruising.

I have witnessed the amazing benefits of ozone water firsthand. My education in kinesiology has allowed me to recognize that ozone water will change the way we treat sports injuries, prepare our food, and stay healthy.

There is absolutely nothing dangerous about ozone water. The benefits are undeniable. TRY IT, and you will agree that Ozone Water Is A Miracle!

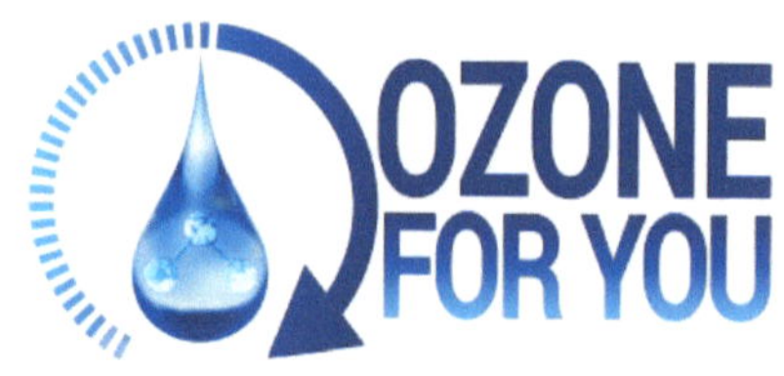

Contact Mike Casey at Ozone For You for consultation and to order your units.

Mike@OzoneForYou.com

714-451-2700